PROSTATE MASSAGE

The Complete Guide With Basic Tips And Techniques On How To Do Prostate Massage Correctly To Improve Sexual Performance And Be Free From all kind of prostate problem

Muller XCrus

Table of Contents

Chapter 1 3
    PROSTATE MASSAGE 3

Chapter 2 6
    WHAT IS PROSTATITIS? 6
    SIGNS OF PROSTATITIS 7
    RISKS 8
    THE BEST TECHNIQUE TO DO A PROSTATE MASSAGE 10

Chapter 3 14
    WHAT ARE THE UPSIDES OF PROSTATE MASSAGE TREATMENT? 14
    WHAT'S IN STORE DURING A PROSTATE MASSAGE 18

Chapter 4 21
    TIPS AND STRATEGIES 21
    THE END 26

Chapter 1

PROSTATE MASSAGE

Prostate back rub is a strategy where a finger is inserted into the rectum to empower the prostate organ. The goal is to convey excess unique fluid the fluid that mixes in with sperm to make semen from the channels of the prostate organ. This therapy might offer some clinical benefits, or your PCP might use it to investigate an issue. In any case, it's not something experts typically recommend or use for testing or treatment. The prostate is a little organ about the size of a golf ball between the establishment of the penis and the rectum. Its major occupation is to make the fluid, in like manner called semen, that helps sperm with journeying and persevere. Massaging the prostate releases that fluid out of your prostate lines To do the system, your PCP will slide a gloved finger into your rectum, then back rub or push on the prostate starting there. It may feel fairly abnormal, yet it doesn't take long. A couple of individuals use standard prostate back rubs to deal direct signs of prostate issues. Experts might play out this using their hands or with a prostate working device. Prostate back rub can be hardly anguishing. A couple of gathering report an extended devouring sensation after squander, due to the substance of the fluids. External prostate back rub may incorporate applying strain on the perineum, the district somewhere close to the backside and the scrotum. Experts can moreover perform prostate back rub by carefully scouring the stomach, between the pubic bone and the gut button. Contraptions are moreover available to assist with outside prostate back rub.

Chapter 2

WHAT IS PROSTATITIS?

Prostatitis is developing and aggravation of the prostate organ. It can cause indications like torture when you pee and torture around your groin and pelvis. An expert might do a prostate back rub to examine the condition. They can test the fluid that comes from your prostate channels to see what's causing the issue. Yet the most broadly perceived medications for prostatitis are immunizing agents poisons and non-steroidal quieting drugs (NSAIDs), prostate back rub is another decision. It can help ease with convincing and extending by conveying fluids that advancement in the prostate. Little assessments have found that plying the area a couple of times every week - close by taking immunizing agents poisons - can give lightening from torture and squeezing factor.

SIGNS OF PROSTATITIS

The signs of prostatitis include:

* Frequent, anguishing, frail, impeded, or deficient pee

* Blood in the pee

* Erectile brokenness

* Painful release

* Fever

* Muscle torture

* Back torture

* Pain close by between the butt and the scrotum.

Irritation of the prostate organ has a couple of causes, including:

* Bacteria

* Non-bacterial microorganisms

* Immune system response

* Nerve hurt

RISKS

The strategy passes on different risks, including:

* making exceptional prostatitis more unfortunate and possibly causing blood hurting, due to a risk of spreading pollution

* Bleeding around the prostate

* Cellulitis, certified skin defilement

* Hemorrhoids flare-ups

* Spreading of prostate illness, on the off chance that it is currently present

* Damage to the rectal covering

THE BEST TECHNIQUE TO DO A PROSTATE MASSAGE

The prostate is a walnut assessed organ inside the rectum and just under the bladder. It folds over the urethra, which is the chamber that channels pee from the bladder. The prostate will overall get greater with age, simplifying it to discover. To find the prostate an individual can install a lubed up finger into the rectum, then push hardly on the front mass of the rectum. They may feel a slight knot. It is furthermore possible to stimulate the prostate less straight by pushing up on the skin between the balls and the rectum, a district called the perineum. Since the prostate is so close to the bladder and urethra, unprecedented prostate induction can make the longing pee. Prostatitis and other prostate issues may in like manner brief more nonstop pee. If performing prostate back rub for sexual purposes, it routinely helps with achieving a state of energy first. Doing as such moves the organ into a fairly up and in invert circumstance as the penis becomes erect. By then, at that point:

* Apply lube liberally around the butt.

* Insert an index finger step by step to the primary knuckle and start jolting off.

* Pull the finger out and re-apply lube.

* As you continue to jolt off, override your finger indeed into the backside, this chance to the ensuing knuckle.

* Repeat stages 3 and 4 until you show up at the third knuckle.

* Once the finger is totally implanted, search for a changed bunch around 4 slithers inside the rectum and up towards the

establishment of the penis. This is the prostate.

* Gently back focus on the prostate a round or forward and backward development using the pile of a finger. You can moreover apply fragile squeezing factor for seven to 10 seconds, again with the heap of a finger rather than the tip.

Chapter 3

WHAT ARE THE UPSIDES OF PROSTATE MASSAGE TREATMENT?

Prostatic back rub is thought to help with clearing the prostatic conductor. This channel, or pipeline, runs between your prostate and the rest of your regenerative and urinary structure. Working might make an unconstrained release of fluid. This emanation may help with getting this line liberated from any fluids. This could help with killing any signs you're experiencing. Clinical investigation disclosures don't comprehensively maintain the use of prostate back rub. Most reports of prostate back rub's benefits are described or result from little case studies. An enormous piece of these reports need more conspicuous evaluation before they can be used as standard clinical direction. Most studies that have looked at the usage of prostate back rub have been small and not conclusive. Subsequently, a couple of experts may not help the usage of prostate back rub. In any case, certain social events of men may benefit from prostate back rub. Men with the going with conditions may find interesting lightening when they use prostate back rub:

* Agonizing release: Back rub treatment may ease fluid blockages in your regenerative structure. These wrinkles may make you experience bother or anguish while releasing. Back rub might kill them.

* Erectile brokenness: Before the present more current treatment options, men used back rub treatment and prostate impelling to treat erectile brokenness (ED). A couple of men really use it today close by other ED prescriptions or alone. More standard ED drugs

fuse remedies, siphons, and installs.

* Pee stream: The prostate envelops your urethra. As extending and disturbance in the prostate augmentation, the prostate may begin to intrude with or even eliminate your movement of pee. If prostate back rub treatment kills a piece of that growing, your pee stream may improve.

* Prostatitis: Prior to against disease specialists and more explicit prescriptions were available, massage treatment was the fundamental treatment for

prostatitis. Since experts grasp a bit more about the gigantic number of issues that make up the prostatitis examination, meds have gotten more explicit.

WHAT'S IN STORE DURING A PROSTATE MASSAGE

A prostate back rub is an incredible arrangement like a modernized rectal test (DRE). Urologists consistently use DREs to check the prostate for bunches, changes, or various signs of possible harmful development. Your PCP may play out a DRE to gain an imparted prostatic emanation that can be furthermore reviewed for signs of prostatitis, tainting, or various issues. During a prostate back rub, the individual playing out the back rub will implant a gloved, lubed up finger into your rectum. They'll carefully go on, or work, the prostate for a couple of moments. In case this back rub is anguishing, tell the individual preforming the back rub. The back rub might be off-kilter a few seconds, anyway it shouldn't be anguishing. How from time to time you have a prostate back rub is reliant upon you and your PCP or the treating capable. You can expect to go to a couple of gatherings consistently for somewhere near a month.

Then, you may have the choice to decrease the amount of visits.

Chapter 4

TIPS AND STRATEGIES

* Use a glove: Before embeddings a finger into the rectum and searching for your (or your assistant's) prostate, slip on an extra latex glove (or vinyl in the event that you're delicate to latex). The glove not simply goes probably as a real obstacle to keep tiny life forms from the hands being brought into the rectal passage, anyway its smooth external will simplify the collaboration by allowing the finger to drift inside. A glove moreover keeps your fingernails

from unexpectedly tearing the touchy skin of the rectum.

* Use lube: A huge piece of prostate depleting is oil. The butt-driven section isn't good for making its own oil, and accordingly you need to give nature some help. Pick a silicone-based lube exceptionally shaped for butt-driven sex, as these will be thicker and longer-persevering.

* Enliven the penis: To build the sensations and release up the rectum, have a go at shocking off all the while as you or your associate examine your prostate. This can moreover extend the

potential outcomes that you'll show up at peak. If you like having a "pure" prostate peak, yet it feels unnecessarily hard, you can strengthen your penis and prostate all the while until you're astoundingly close topping. Presently, quit reaching your penis and spotlight totally on the prostate until you tip over the edge.

* Enlist an accessory: In the occasion that you've never examined your own prostate, it might feel easier to have the help of an accessory as you get your bearing. Combining prostate back rub into your sexual conjunction

can be a lovely strategy to unite both of you. The impression of being reached from inside by someone you trust is incredibly close.

* Use a sex toy: If you feel a little nauseous about putting your finger inside yourself, you can enlist the help of a twisted dildo to help with showing up at your prostate. Post for dildos that are recorded as being outlined to hit "the P-spot." You can in like manner get dildos that vibrate; this can add an extra layer of capacity to your prostate examinations.

* Take a full breath: In the event that you're not used to exploring your butt, it can feel to some degree frightening consistently. Guarantee that you're in a calm setting, with a ton of time set aside. Faint the lights, take heaps of full breaths in through your nose and out of your mouth, and take the necessary steps not to stress as you examine. While you might be captivated to two or three drinks to work with the cycle, it's enormously improved to focus in on your breathing since in the event that you're intoxicated you may inadvertently hurt yourself.

THE END